Table of Contents

Introduction

Antibiotic resistance is the ability of a microorganism to withstand the effects of an antibiotic.

It is a specific type of drug resistance.

Antibiotic resistance evolves naturally via natural selection through random mutation, but it could also be engineered by applying an evolutionary stress on a population.

Once such a gene is generated, bacteria can then transfer the genetic information in a horizontal fashion (between individuals) by plasmid exchange.

If a bacterium carries several resistance genes, it is called multiresistant or, informally, a superbug.

Causes Antibiotic resistance can also be introduced artificially into a microorganism through transformation protocols.

This can be a useful way of implanting artificial genes into the microorganism.

Antibiotic resistance is a consequence of evolution via natural selection.

The antibiotic action is an environmental pressure; those bacteria which have a mutation allowing them to survive will live on to reproduce.

They will then pass this trait to their offspring, which will be a fully resistant generation.

Several studies have demonstrated that patterns of antibiotic usage greatly affect the number of resistant organisms which develop.

Overuse of broad-spectrum antibiotics, such as second- and third-generation cephalosporins, greatly hastens the development of methicillin resistance.

Other factors contributing towards resistance include incorrect diagnosis, unnecessary prescriptions, improper use of antibiotics by patients, and the use of antibiotics as livestock food additives for growth promotion.

Researchers have recently demonstrated the bacterial protein LexA may play a key role in the acquisition of bacterial mutations.

Resistant pathogens Staphylococcus aureus (colloquially known as "Staph aureus" or a Staph infection) is one of the major resistant pathogens.

Found on the mucous membranes and the skin of around a third of the population, it is extremely adaptable to antibiotic pressure.

It was the first bacterium in which penicillin resistance was found—in 1947, just four years after the drug started being mass-produced.

Methicillin was then the antibiotic of choice, but has since been replaced by oxacillin due to significant kidney toxicity.

MRSA (methicillin-resistant Staphylococcus aureus) was first detected in Britain in 1961 and is now "quite common" in hospitals.

MRSA was responsible for 37% of fatal cases of blood poisoning in the UK in 1999, up from 4% in 1991.

Half of all S. aureus infections in the US are resistant to penicillin, methicillin, tetracycline and erythromycin.

This left vancomycin as the only effective agent available at the time.

However, strains with intermediate (4-8 ug/ml) levels of resistence, termed GISA (glycopeptide intermediate Staphylococcus aureus) or VISA (vancomycin intermediate Staphylococcus aureus), began appearing the the late 1990s.

The first identified case was in Japan in 1996, and strains have since been found in hospitals in England, France and the US.

The first documented strain with complete (>16ug/ml) resistence to vancomycin, termed VRSA (Vancomycin-resistant Staphylococcus aureus) appeared in the United States in 2002.

A new class of antibiotics, oxazolidinones, became available in the 1990s, and the first commercially available oxazolidinone, linezolid, is comparable to vancomycin in effectiveness against MRSA.

Linezolid-resistance in Staphylococcus aureus was reported in 2003.

CA-MRSA (Community-acquired MRSA) has now emerged as an epidemic that is responsible for rapidly progressive, fatal diseases including necrotizing pneumonia, severe sepsis and necrotizing fasciitis.

Methicillin-resistant Staphylococcus aureus (MRSA) is the most frequently identified antimicrobial drug-resistant pathogen in US hospitals.

The epidemiology of infections caused by MRSA is rapidly changing.

In the past 10 years, infections caused by this organism have emerged in the community.

The 2 MRSA clones in the United States most closely associated with community outbreaks, USA400 (MW2 strain, ST1 lineage) and USA300, often contain Panton-Valentine leukocidin (PVL) genes and, more frequently, have been associated with skin and soft tissue infections.

Outbreaks of community-associated (CA)-MRSA infections have been reported in correctional facilities, among athletic teams, among military recruits, in newborn nurseries, and among active homosexual men.

CA-MRSA infections now appear to be endemic in many urban regions and cause most CA-S. aureus infections.

Enterococcus faecium is another superbug found in hospitals.

Penicillin-Resistant Enterococcus was seen in 1983, Vancomycin-Resistant Enterococcus (VRE) in 1987, and Linezolid-Resistant Enterococcus (LRE) in the late 1990s.

Streptococcus pyogenes (Group A Streptococcus: GAS) infections can usually be treated with many different antibiotics.

Early treatment may reduce the risk of death from invasive group A streptococcal disease.

However, even the best medical care does not prevent death in every case.

For those with very severe illness, supportive care in an intensive care unit may be needed.

For persons with necrotizing fasciitis, surgery often is needed to remove damaged tissue.

Strains of S. pyogenes resistant to macrolide antibiotics have emerged, however all strains remain uniformly sensitive to penicillin.

Resistance of Streptococcus pneumoniae to penicillin and other beta-lactams is increasing worldwide.

The major mechanism of resistance involves the introduction of mutations in genes encoding penicillin-binding proteins.

Selective pressure is thought to play an important role, and use of beta-lactam antibiotics has been implicated as a risk factor for infection and colonization.

Streptococcus pneumoniae is responsible for pneumonia, bacteremia, otitis media, meningitis, sinusitis, peritonitis and arthritis.

Introduction

Antibiotics are medicines used to prevent and treat bacterial infections. Antibiotic resistance occurs when bacteria change in response to the use of these medicines.

Bacteria, not humans or animals, become antibiotic-resistant. These bacteria may infect humans and animals, and the infections they cause are harder to treat than those caused by non-resistant bacteria.

Antibiotic resistance leads to higher medical costs, prolonged hospital stays, and increased mortality.

The world urgently needs to change the way it prescribes and uses antibiotics. Even if new medicines are developed, without behaviour change, antibiotic resistance will remain a major threat. Behaviour changes must also include actions to reduce the spread of infections through vaccination, hand washing, practising safer sex, and good food hygiene.

Scope of the problem

Antibiotic resistance is rising to dangerously high levels in all parts of the world. New resistance mechanisms are emerging and spreading globally, threatening our ability to treat common infectious diseases. A growing list of infections – such as pneumonia, tuberculosis, blood poisoning, gonorrhoea, and foodborne diseases – are becoming harder, and sometimes impossible, to treat as antibiotics become less effective.

Where antibiotics can be bought for human or animal use without a prescription, the emergence and spread of resistance is made worse. Similarly, in countries without standard treatment guidelines, antibiotics are often over-prescribed by health workers and veterinarians and over-used by the public.

Without urgent action, we are heading for a post-antibiotic era, in which common infections and minor injuries can once again kill.

Prevention and control

Antibiotic resistance is accelerated by the misuse and overuse of antibiotics, as well as poor infection prevention and control. Steps can be taken at all levels of society to reduce the impact and limit the spread of resistance.

Individuals

To prevent and control the spread of antibiotic resistance, individuals can:

• Only use antibiotics when prescribed by a certified health professional.

• Never demand antibiotics if your health worker says you don't need them.

• Always follow your health worker's advice when using antibiotics.

• Never share or use leftover antibiotics.

• Prevent infections by regularly washing hands, preparing food hygienically, avoiding close contact with sick people, practising safer sex, and keeping vaccinations up to date.

• Prepare food hygienically, following the WHO Five Keys to Safer Food (keep clean, separate raw and cooked, cook thoroughly, keep food at safe temperatures, use safe water and raw materials) and choose foods that have been produced without the use of antibiotics for growth promotion or disease prevention in healthy animals.

Policy makers

To prevent and control the spread of antibiotic resistance, policy makers can:

• Ensure a robust national action plan to tackle antibiotic resistance is in place.

• Improve surveillance of antibiotic-resistant infections.

- Strengthen policies, programmes, and implementation of infection prevention and control measures.

- Regulate and promote the appropriate use and disposal of quality medicines.

- Make information available on the impact of antibiotic resistance.

Health professionals

To prevent and control the spread of antibiotic resistance, health professionals can:

- Prevent infections by ensuring your hands, instruments, and environment are clean.

• Only prescribe and dispense antibiotics when they are needed, according to current guidelines.

• Report antibiotic-resistant infections to surveillance teams.

• Talk to your patients about how to take antibiotics correctly, antibiotic resistance and the dangers of misuse.

• Talk to your patients about preventing infections (for example, vaccination, hand washing, safer sex, and covering nose and mouth when sneezing).

Healthcare industry

To prevent and control the spread of antibiotic resistance, the health industry can:

• Invest in research and development of new antibiotics, vaccines, diagnostics and other tools.

Agriculture sector

To prevent and control the spread of antibiotic resistance, the agriculture sector can:

• Only give antibiotics to animals under veterinary supervision.

• Not use antibiotics for growth promotion or to prevent diseases in healthy animals.

• Vaccinate animals to reduce the need for antibiotics and use alternatives to antibiotics when available.

• Promote and apply good practices at all steps of production and processing of foods from animal and plant sources.

• Improve biosecurity on farms and prevent infections through improved hygiene and animal welfare.

Recent developments

While there are some new antibiotics in development, none of them are expected to be effective against the most dangerous forms of antibiotic-resistant bacteria.

Given the ease and frequency with which people now travel, antibiotic resistance is a global problem, requiring efforts from all nations and many sectors.

Impact

When infections can no longer be treated by first-line antibiotics, more expensive medicines must be used. A longer duration of illness and treatment, often in hospitals, increases health care costs as well as the economic burden on families and societies.

Antibiotic resistance is putting the achievements of modern medicine at risk. Organ transplantations, chemotherapy and surgeries such as caesarean sections become much more dangerous without effective antibiotics for the prevention and treatment of infections.

WHO response

Tackling antibiotic resistance is a high priority for WHO. A global action plan on antimicrobial resistance, including antibiotic resistance, was endorsed at the World Health Assembly in May 2015. The global action plan aims to ensure prevention and treatment of infectious diseases with safe and effective medicines.

The "Global action plan on antimicrobial resistance" has 5 strategic objectives:

- To improve awareness and understanding of antimicrobial resistance.

- To strengthen surveillance and research.

- To reduce the incidence of infection.

• To optimize the use of antimicrobial medicines.

• To ensure sustainable investment in countering antimicrobial resistance.

A political declaration endorsed by Heads of State at the United Nations General Assembly in New York in September 2016 signaled the world's commitment to taking a broad, coordinated approach to address the root causes of antimicrobial resistance across multiple sectors, especially human health, animal health and agriculture. WHO is supporting Member States to develop national action plans on antimicrobial resistance, based on the global action plan.

WHO has been leading multiple initiatives to address **antimicrobial resistance:**

World Antibiotic Awareness Week

Held every November since 2015 with the theme "Antibiotics: Handle with care", the global, multi-year campaign has increasing volume of activities during the week of the campaign.

The Global Antimicrobial Resistance Surveillance System (GLASS)

The WHO-supported system supports a standardized approach to the collection, analysis and sharing of data related to antimicrobial resistance at a global level to inform decision-making, drive local, national and regional action.

Global Antibiotic Research and Development Partnership (GARDP)

A joint initiative of WHO and Drugs for Neglected Diseases initiative (DNDi), GARDP encourages research and development through public-private partnerships. By 2023, the partnership aims to develop and deliver up to four new treatments, through improvement of existing antibiotics and acceleration of the entry of new antibiotic drugs.

Interagency Coordination Group on Antimicrobial Resistance (IACG)

The United Nations Secretary-General has established IACG to improve coordination between international organizations and to ensure effective global action against this threat to health security. The IACG is co-chaired by the UN Deputy Secretary-General and the Director General of WHO and comprises high level representatives of relevant UN agencies, other international organizations, and individual experts across different sectors.

Fast Facts

Facts about Antibiotic Resistance

• Antibiotic resistance is one of the most urgent threats to the public's health.

- Every time a person takes antibiotics, sensitive bacteria are killed, but resistant ones may be left to grow and multiply.

- Overuse of antibiotics is a major cause of increases in drug-resistant bacteria.

- Overuse and misuse of antibiotics threatens the usefulness of these important drugs. Decreasing inappropriate antibiotic use is a key strategy to control antibiotic resistance.

- Antibiotic resistance in children and older adults is of particular concern because these age groups have the highest rates of antibiotic use.

• Antibiotic resistance can cause significant suffering for people who have common infections that once were easily treatable with antibiotics.

• When antibiotics do not work, infections often last longer, cause more severe illness, require more doctor visits or longer hospital stays, and involve more expensive and toxic medications. Some resistant infections can even cause death.

CBD and Antibiotics

CBD has been widely known for its array of medicinal benefits ranging from Epilepsy, to cancer, to arthritis. Not much has been researched on the topic of CBD and antibiotic resistance, but here I will piece together everything I could find about

CBD, its antibacterial properties, as well as antibiotics as a whole.

How Do Antibiotics Work?

Antibiotics were established in 1928 with the discover of penicillin by Alexander Fleming.

He found that antibiotics work by affecting human cells in a way that is specific to bacterial cells. Allowing us to gain the same protection that bacteria do from diseases.

For example, antibiotics have a cell wall, where human cells don't. When you take penicillin, it keeps the bacteria from building a cell wall, allowing human cells to fight them off more easily. Antibiotics also play a role in slowing protein building and DNA copying for certain bacterial cells.

How does CBD work?

CBD works by affecting the endocannabinoid system using neurotransmitters called cannabinoids. Our bodies naturally produce these chemicals and CBD indirectly stimulates these neurons. After which it produces an array of sensations and medicinal benefits.

To learn more about CBD and its effects on the brain and body, check out my earlier post here

CBD and Antibiotics Research

Not much research has been done on CBD and antibiotics, but there has been some indirect work to understand their relationship. Almost 60% of all pharmaceutical drugs, including antibiotics are processed by the liver through a family of enzymes called P450.

These same P450 enzymes are used to metabolize CBD, and is the reason why there could potentially be interactions with antibiotics. As CBD goes into the liver it starts utilizing all the P450 and it metabolizing capability. This could limit P450s availability in being able to break down other drugs that rely on the same enzyme. Not to say that the other drugs don't get metabolized, but they do so a lot slower, or in a different fashion.

Apart from just CBD, other things have this same effect on the P450 enzymes, such a grapefruit. You may have been told by your doctor not to eat grapefruit while taking a specific medication, and this is the reason why. CBD is thought to be a much stronger P450 enzyme inhibitor than grapefruit and should be something to think about what taking CBD and antibiotics. More research is needed to fully understand this relationship, but it can be said with confidence that CBD does utilize the same breakdown enzymes as antibiotics.

Are All Antibiotics Broken Down This Way?

No! Only Macrolide antibiotics are broken down by the P450 enzyme, so they are the ones of concern when taking CBD. These types of antibiotics are commonly prescribed for respiratory tract and skin infections.

Examples of Macrolide Antibiotics

o Azithromycin

o Clarithromycin

o Erythromycin

o Spiramycin

o Telithromycin

There are potentially other medications that classify and Macrolide antibiotics, but this is just a short list of some that I found. Make sure to ask your doctor if you want to know for sure.

How do Macrolide Antibiotics Work?

Macrolide antibiotics work by affecting ribosomes, which are the protein building machines of the cells. Ribosomes are responsible for building proteins in bother human and bacterial cells, but there are some differences.

The main difference is that Macrolides prevent bacterial cells from building proteins by blocking their ribosomes. This makes it so the bacterial cells can't build protein and thus can't survive.

Should I be worried taking CBD with Antibiotics?

If you are taking antibiotics that are treating your respiratory tract or a skin infection, then there is some cause to think twice about taking CBD. There probably won't be to harmful of consequences, but the CBD and antibiotic interactions could keep your medications from working properly. This could negatively affect your health if you strongly need the antibiotics to survive. Make sure to fully understand the types of medications you are taking before thinking of combining CBD and antibiotics.

Taking CBD and Antibiotics Together

If your considering taking CBD and antibiotics together, consult your doctor and see what they have to say. CBD can be used to treat a variety of different symptoms, so it can be understood why someone taking antibiotics might also want to take CBD. The most important thing when wondering about drug interactions is to talk to your doctor first.

CBD Oil vs Antibiotics – Cannabis or Over the Counter Drugs?

The discovery of antibiotics as a medicine in 1928 meant only a huge revolution in health care. Nevertheless, the production and universal use of antibiotics rapidly increased in the period preceding the end of World War II, and this excessive consumption of antibiotics in humans changed to today's sad reality, as if by a magic wand.

Spend some time reading Healthy Hemp Oil Reviews and save yourself from troubles buying a bad brand. Anyways let's continue.

According to a recent report by the Center for Disease Control (CDC), about half of prescriptions for antibiotics are completely unnecessary in the US. According to another report of the World Health Organization (WHO), the impact of excessive consumption of antibiotics is directly catastrophic. And the bacteria that are usually present in the human body, constantly develop and strengthen the immunity to the multitude of antibiotics that people usually use for diseases, and cannot even be classified as serious.

Antibiotics and the consequences of their excessive use

This catastrophe is better explained by statistics, which states that at least 2 million Americans suffer from an infection each year caused by increased immunity to bacteria. It is estimated that about 23 000 deaths.

If this problem is not rectified on time, the number of these deaths can increase rapidly in the coming years. But the good news is that nature has already found a solution to this problem.

A study of the endurance and resistance of bacteria to CBD

Studies of British and Italian scientists have shown that CCD has a natural potential for the effective destruction of these bacteria and is therefore very effective in the treatment of infections.

At least 6 of the most resistant bacteria were exposed to CBD, and fortunately, in all cases, CBD oil proved to be much more effective in controlling resistant bacteria than any drug available in the pharmacy.

Cannabidiol and its antimicrobial effects

It was also found that CCD oil should be applied sublingually to make the effect as effective as possible (through the oral mucosa). These antimicrobial effects of CBD, which are absorbed by the mucosa in the body, are very effective in fighting these resistant bacteria and their infection.

It follows that cannabis, which is not normally used for recreational purposes, can be used to develop effective medicines for patients at an affordable price. Thus, CBD can be a substance that treats and is effective and accessible to patients.

Manufacture of drugs with CBD

Given all of the above, it is easy to conclude that CBD is the most effective drug for treating infection caused by bacteria resistant to antibiotics. The final step in the development of effective CBC drugs is obtaining permission from the US government to promote and use cannabidiol.

Although this seems to be a complex and endless process, considering all the advantages that CBD offers for fighting bacterial infections, it is likely that soon cannabidiol will be approved as an effective drug for patients.

CBD as a Superbug Antibiotic?

June 24, 2019 -- Cannabidiol, or CBD, already being researched and used for anxiety, insomnia, epilepsy and pain, may be the next superbug fighter for resistant infections, a new study suggests.

The researchers tested CBD against a wide variety of bacteria, "including bacteria that have become resistant to the most commonly used antibiotics," says Mark Blaskovich, PhD, senior research officer at the Centre for Superbug Solutions at the Institute for Molecular Bioscience at the University of Queensland in Australia.

The development is important, as antibiotic resistance is reaching dangerously high levels, according to the World Health Organization.

What the Research Shows

CBD is a non-psychoactive compound taken from cannabis and hemp; it does not produce the high that regular marijuana does. To date, the FDA has only approved CBD for treating rare and severe forms of seizure, although it is promoted for many other health benefits.

Blaskovich presented the research Sunday at the American Society for Microbiology annual meeting. The research includes work in test tubes and animal models. Research presented at meetings should be viewed as preliminary until published in a peer-reviewed medical journal.

"The first thing we looked at is CBD's ability to kill bacteria," he says. "In every case, CBD had a very similar potency to that of common antibiotics."

The researchers tested the CBD against some strains of staphylococcus, which cause skin infections, and streptococcus, which cause strep throat.

They compared how effective CBD was compared to common antibiotics, such as vancomycin and daptomycin. "We looked at how quickly the CBD killed the bacteria. It's quite fast, within 3 hours, which is pretty good. Vancomycin (Vancocin) kills over 6 to 8 hours."

The CBD also disrupted the biofilm, the layer of "goop" around bacteria that makes it more difficult for the antibiotic to penetrate and kill.

Finally, the lab studies showed that "CBD is much less likely to cause resistance than the existing antibiotics," Blaskovich says.

The CBD "is selective for the type of bacteria," he says.

He found it effective against gram-positive bacteria but not gram-negative. Gram-positive bacteria cause serious skin infections and pneumonia, among other conditions. Gram-negative bacteria include salmonella (found in undercooked foods) and E. coli (the cause of urinary tract infections, diarrhea, and other ailments), among other bacteria.

In another study, also presented at the meeting, the researchers tested topical

CBD to treat a skin infection on mice. It cut the number of bacteria after 48 hours, Blaskovich says, although it did not clear the infection. That research is ongoing.

How It Might Work, Caveats

The researchers can't say exactly how the CBD may prove to be a superbug infection fighter. "We thought it might work by damaging the outer membrane of the bacteria, to make it leaky," Blaskovich says. "It doesn't seem to do that. It might be a completely new mechanism of action."

He says the research results are promising but in early stages. He also warns people that it's much too early to self-treat infections with CBD.

The study was funded by Botanix Pharmaceuticals Ltd., which is researching uses of CBD for skin conditions, and the Australian government. Blaskovich is a consultant for Botanix.

Perspective

Brandon Novy, a microbiology researcher at Reed College in Portland, OR, calls the study findings "very promising," since the results show the bacteria were not able to form resistance to the CBD, and since the bacteria were not able to form a biofilm.

All About CBD Oil

What Is CBD?

It's short for cannabidiol, and it's a natural compound found in both marijuana and hemp plants. There's some evidence that it might help treat pain, seizures, and some other health problems. But much more research is needed for doctors to know for sure what it can do.

How Do You Take It?

You can take CBD oil by itself by mouth, or use one of many products that has it as an ingredient. These include pills, chewable gels, "tinctures" you drop under your tongue, vape cartridges you breathe in, creams on your skin, and foods like chocolate bars. The amount and quality of CBD in these products can be very different.

Does It Make You High?

CBD doesn't -- another substance in marijuana called THC does that. If you use a CBD product, check the label and make sure that's the only cannabinoid listed. In states where marijuana is legal, some companies put product information online that lists the amount of each ingredient.

Is It Addictive?

CBD oil by itself is not. But CBD products that also have THC can be. The key again is to know the source and check the ingredients and the amounts so you know exactly what you're using.

Where Is It Legal?

Forty-seven states now allow some form of CBD. Only Idaho, South Dakota, and Nebraska ban all marijuana use. Legal details are different by state, so do your research to make sure you're on the right side of the law.

Can CBD Help With Seizures?

The FDA has approved only one CBD-based drug, and it's used to treat two rare types of epilepsy: Lennox-Gastaut syndrome and Dravet syndrome. It's called Epidiolex, and it's approved for adults and kids over age 2.

Can It Ease Pain?

Scientists are working to see if it might help with arthritis, and some people with HIV say it helps relieve nerve pain (also called neuropathy). There's some evidence that it may help muscle spasms linked to multiple sclerosis, too. More research is needed to know for sure.

Does It Help Blood Pressure?

In normal conditions, CBD doesn't seem to affect this one way or the other. But researchers are studying whether it might help keep your blood pressure stable when you're stressed. More work needs to be done before scientists fully understand its effects.

Does It Help Inflammation?

Early studies show that CBD might help with this, especially if it's related to arthritis, MS, diabetes, or Alzheimer's. But scientists are still trying to prove that and figure out how it works.

Does CBD Help Cancer?

In studies done on lab mice, CBD oil showed promise at killing breast cancer cells and making chemotherapy drugs work better. But researchers have much more work to do to see if CBD can help people in that way.

Is It Good for Your Skin?

There is evidence that CBD might be a treatment for acne. It seems to help with both the inflammation that can lead to breakouts and the amount of fatty acids in the blood, which can make them worse. It also may protect skin cells from damage.

Does It Help Psychosis?

One study showed it helped ease the symptoms of psychosis in people with schizophrenia, but more research is needed to know just how well it might work. Keep in mind that THC, which is found in a number of CBD products, can have the opposite effect, and product labels aren't always accurate.

Does It Help Addiction?

Much more study is needed, but early studies show that CBD may help people who want to break their addiction to cigarettes as well as drugs like heroin, cocaine, and methamphetamine. This may be in part because it seems to help with anxiety and muscle tension.

Are There Side Effects?

So far, CBD doesn't seem to cause serious ones. When it's used to treat epilepsy or psychotic disorders, people reported tiredness, diarrhea, and changes in appetite. But CBD can affect how other medications work, so be sure to tell your doctor about everything you take, including vitamins and supplements.

Both findings are important. "The biofilm is an important part of the whole infection process," he says. "It helps the bacteria attach [to whatever surface or host] and survive."

At the same meeting, Novy presented a preliminary study, finding that CBD also looks promising to fight some gram-negative infections.

"It is an important study that deserves to be followed up on," says Amesh Adalja, MD, an infectious disease doctor and senior scholar at the Johns Hopkins Center for Health Security.

He was not involved in the new study. But he cautions that "it is important to keep it all in context. I think it is a good thing that people are looking at the use of CBD for infectious uses in a systematic way."

But the work so far is only in test tubes and animals. Many question remain, such as looking at whether it is toxic, doses, and the best way to deliver the CBD, Adalja says. He, too, cautions against self-treating with CBD for infections.

Summary

Antibiotics are medicines that fight bacterial infections. Used properly, they can save lives. But there is a growing problem of antibiotic resistance. It happens when bacteria change and become able to resist the effects of an antibiotic.

Using antibiotics can lead to resistance. Each time you take antibiotics, sensitive bacteria are killed. But resistant germs may be left to grow and multiply. They can spread to other people. They can also cause infections that certain antibiotics cannot cure. Methicillin-resistant Staphylococcus aureus (MRSA) is one example. It causes infections that are resistant to several common antibiotics.

To help prevent antibiotic resistance

• Don't use antibiotics for viruses like colds or flu. Antibiotics don't work on viruses.

• Don't pressure your doctor to give you an antibiotic.

• When you take antibiotics, follow the directions carefully. Finish your medicine even if you feel better. If you stop treatment too soon, some bacteria may survive and re-infect you.

- Don't save antibiotics for later or use someone else's prescription.